THE HERBAL SURVIVAL GUIDEBOOK

By Reverend Dr. Donia Gonzales-Copeland

2 Covenant Mogul Publishing

Theeaglerealm.org

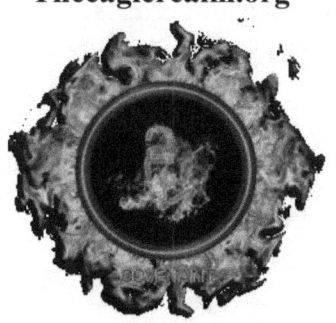

The Herbal Survival Guidebook

The Herbalist Survivors Guide

For Beginner Users

By Dr. Donia Gonzales-Copeland MA. DPC.

©2015 Donia Gonzales-Copeland

Project Manager: 2 Covenant Mogul

Cover Artist: 2 Covenant Mogul

Editor: Donia Gonzales-Copeland

Printed in the United States of America. Published By:

2 Covenant Mogul Publishing LLC Utilizing Microsoft

Publishing Software. Websites CPR and Emergency Training Online, Herbal First Aid Books, and Sites Basic Herbal Preparations Simpler Method.

Resources from Renewal of the Spirit Institute

Note: for anyone seeking information about resources, books, herbal products, vitamins, organizations, schools and alternative health. Please contact Dr. Donia Gonzales-Copeland at 302-834-5407, renewalof48@yahoo.com or gcopelandd@aol.com

Renewal of the Spirit Institute conducts classes on herbs, aromatherapy, reiki touch healing, and Pastoral Counseling. We offer certificates and diplomas through a reputable interfaith seminary.

Please contact us for information about our school, or visit us on line at:

www.renewalofthespiritinstitute.com

We have classes, correspondence courses, and online courses.

Dedication

This book is dedicated to my husband Iszell Copeland, Jr.,
My Daughter' Serena, Terri & Aisha. My son Joseph, My
granddaughter's Diamond, Amira, Hadiya, Arianna & my
grandson Amir. My great granddaughters Angel & Ari.
And my best friend Sandra.

The Herbal Survival Guidebook

Contents

Chapters

One..................................Preparing Your

72 Hour Kit

Chapter Two - The Foods Your Family Will Need

Chapter Three.........The Emergency Herbal

Medicine Chest

Chapter Four..................Teaching Yourself

First Aid

The Herbal Survival Guidebook

INTRODUCTON

This book is not to scare you but to help you be prepared for any disaster. I woke up one day to my Awaken Spiritual Self and I discovered all the thing I already knew should be written down & taught. So here I am.

I am the founder of Renewal of the Spirit Institute & Wholistic Center. The school was founded for those seeking to follow God's call to the ministry and to work independently with God's plan for them. The school provides Training in Pastoral Counseling, HIV Training, Domestic Violence Training, Reiki, Hospice Training, Theology the Institute also provides herbal training, holistic health care training, Life Mapping, and also has a healing school.

Well hurry up and turn the page into some fun and excitement, you should find everything you need. This book will be fun and informative for the entire family.

1 PETER 5:8-9 (NIV)

[8] Be alert and of sober mind. Your enemy the devil prowls around like a roaring lion looking for someone to devour. [9] Resist him, standing firm in the faith, because you know that the family of believers throughout the world is undergoing the same kind of sufferings.

Chapter 1

Preparing Your 72 Hour Kit

It is in your best interest to prepare a **72 hour kit.** It should be placed in a location in your house where you can have easy access, should an emergency arise. Remember when an emergency of any type occurs you will not have to go around your house to collect the items you will need.

I suggest you take the time along the family members to gather up whatever you need to survive for at least 3 days. Your items should be collected and stored in a safe place by your front, back, or side door.

What should you pack? You should pack your birth certificate, insurance papers, deeds, bank accounts and recent deposit statements. Loan statements with numbers, securities, copies of your mortgage bill/s, marriage certificate, social security cards, driver's license, medical and dental records. A list of boats, cars, trucks, and campers you may own, and any other important papers that are necessary. Pack all your paper items in plastic Ziploc bags. This will keep them dry and airtight. Make sure that you keep a list of the dates that certain paper work may need to be updated, i.e. medication, driver's license, insurance, etc.

Pack suitcases with changes of clothes, shoes, underwear, socks, diapers, wash cloths, towels, soap, toothpaste, toothbrushes, deodorant, lotion, aspirin, band aids, alcohol, peroxide, witch hazel, hand sanitizer, liquid soap, wet wipes,

Bug spray, blankets, sleeping bags, pillows, flashlights, batteries, coats, sweaters, hats, gloves, rain gear, and soap powder, metal or plastics basins for washing out cloths. Matches, lighters, lighter fluid, charcoal, starter fluid, barbeque pit, garbage bags, hunting knife, and Swiss knife, hunting rifle, mirror, comb, brush, money in small bills, and change. Razors, lip balm, sunscreen, feminine products, bandanas, waterless soap/shampoo, portable radios, ammunition, candles, sterno, butane stoves, a first aid kit, an inflatable raft or some sort of canoe for flood situations.

Some kind of helpful things can be a magnifying glass which you can hold near sun light and over paper to start a fire.

Remember all emergency supplies should be ready in case of any kind of disaster.

Suit Cases and Containers

The best type of suit cases should actually be containers. It should have band aids, gauze, butterfly band aids, cotton balls, small rolls of gauze, various types of tape, cotton swabs, safety pins, cold packs, smelling salts, alcohol swabs, eyedroppers, Benadryl, aspirin, peroxide, wet wipes, Aleve, scissors, thermometers, a crushable heat pack, chewable children's aspirin or Tylenol, cough syrup adult's and children's, packets of antiseptic creams, antiseptic wipes for cuts and scrapes. Pins, needles, threads, safety pins, yarn, knitting needles, materials for patching things. Anti-itch spray, wipes, or cream for bug bites, poison ivy, oak, etc. Toilet paper, Kleenex, napkins, hand warmers, compass, at least 50 feet or more of nylon cord, various sizes of plastic bags. All Medications and Epi-pens.

What to Pack

For children and infants you need to assemble items like diapers (cloth), infant milk, powered milk, powered cocoa mix, baby food, baby wipes, at least six to eight changes of cloths, keep their items separate in a waterproof backpack.

Remember that clothing and footwear should be heavy duty work clothing for both hot and cold weather. Keep an ongoing list of the clothing items you have packed because if you have a growing family their sizes will change. I have been told that wool socks are important to have because they keep your feet warm especially while you sleep.

Car Survival

If you are temporarily stuck in your car you should have a car survival kit. It should consist of flashlights in your glove compartment, under the passenger's seat, in the back of the car and one in the trunk. You should have blankets, if you consistently travel with children you should have one for each child. You need sweater/s, a rain poncho/s, an old heavy coat/s.

Bottles of water, washcloths, towels, paper towels, toilet paper, soap, hand sanitizer, Kleenex, and a well prepared first aid kit. You should also have matches, a battery operated radio, batteries, a hunting knife, Swiss knife, and some non-perishable foods, i.e. crackers, hard candies, dried fruits, instant oatmeal, powdered milk, dried soup, gum, granola bars, instant pudding, powdered drink mixes. These items can be stored in a flat plastic storage bin that you can slide into the trunk of your car. You also can include a can opener and a few sterno cylinders. This could help you if you are trapped in your car and you have to rely on short term shelter.

Survival in Your Own Home

If you are trapped inside your home and cannot leave for reasons like flood, hurricane, etc. You need to prepare yourself even though you are at home. There are still many things you need. Make sure you have flashlights in key locations of your home. Make sure you have extra batteries in those key locations as well. Make sure you have candles and oil lamps in key locations throughout the house, with matches and lighters in place just in case the lights go out.

Always keep sternos handy should you not be able to use your stove can still warm up food on the sterno. I encourage each household to purchase a generator. Keep non-perishable dried foods in place, as well as bottled water, fruits and nuts. Keep phones charged up so that you may be able to use them to call out for help. Drape something out of the window which will let search parties know that you may be trapped inside.

The Closet Use

Keep all emergency kits in all your closets, I heard a women on a talk show say that she was trapped in her closet during one of those mudslides in California. She could not make it all the way in but thanks to her son telling her what to put in the closet, blankets, pillows, etc. She might not have survived.

Shelter Information

Every adult in the house should know where various shelters would be set up in case of emergency. This way your 72 hour kit packed and ready, you can move your family quickly and safely to the shelter.

Fuel (I got this from FEMA and from my Girl Scott days).

Every family member should have fire starting materials and know how to start a fire. Several of these items should be assembled into a kit and labeled as a "fire starting kit." Teach all family members how to use them and let them practice building fires with all methods until they feel totally confident with their ability to do so. Even little children 5 or 6 can be safely instructed in correct fire building techniques under proper supervision. Then if an emergency arises, they will not panic, feel overwhelmed or frightened at the prospect of building a fire for their warmth and protection.

Some different sources are:

- Matches, carry at least two dozen wooden kitchen matches that have been dipped in wax or nail polish to make them waterproof or carry them in a waterproof container.

- Metal match, waterproof, fireproof, durable, and non-toxic. Will light thousands of fires. Available at sporting goods stores.

- Magnesium fire starters are good for starting fires with wet or damp wood. Shave magnesium shavings off a magnesium block with a pocket knife and then strike a spark from a flint with a pocket knife. Magnesium burns exceptionally hot and will ignite almost any combustible material. Works even when wet and can be purchased at most sporting goods stores.

- Small magnifying glass, use to concentrate sunlight onto paper, shredded bark or other tinder.

- Flint and steel a spark from flint steel (such as an empty cigarette lighter or flint and steel striking bar), when directed at dry paper (especially toilet tissue). Shredded bark, dry grass, or other tinder. If patiently persisted will work very well to start a fire. This is the most reliable "non-match" method of starting a fire.

- Commercial fire starter kits, these come in a variety of styles and fuels.

- Steel wool, fine steel wool, (used for scrubbing pots and pans, but not Brillo pads or other types that have soap already impregnated into then) can be used for tinder. Hold two "D" flashlight cells together in one hand (or a 9 volt transistor radio battery) while touching one end of a clump of steel wool to the positive end of the battery and the other end of the steel wool to the negative end of the battery. The current causes the steel wool fibers to incandescent and then produce a flame. It burns very hot and fairly fast so have lots of tinder to burn once the steel wool ignites.

- Candles can be used for warmth, light, and starting fires. To start a fire simply cut a piece of candle about ½ inch in length and place it on top of the tinder. When lit the wax will run over the tinder making it act as a wick and ignite. You can also place small twigs and other easily burnable materials directly into the flame to build a fire.

- Car battery, if you are near a car you can easily put sparks into tinder by attaching any wires to the battery posts and scraping the ends together in the tinder.

- Sterno fuel and stoves make an excellent cooking fuel when backpacking or in emergencies. Sterno can be lit with a match or by a spark from flint and steel. Slivers of gelled sterno can be cut from the can and placed on top of tinder and lit with flint and steel or with a match. It burns hot enough to ignite even damp tinder.

- Cotton balls and gauze from the first aid kit make excellent tinder and can be ignited with sparks or matches.

- Fuel tablets such as tri-oxane and gelled fuels store well and ignite quickly and easily. Some can be fairly expensive.

- Butane and propane stoves, these are made especially for backpackers. The fuel is cheaper than sterno, it burns hotter and it heats better in windy situations than other fuels. Propane however is more difficult to light as outside temperatures near zero.

Tips for Work Survival

We all stand a 40-50% chance of being trapped at work when a tornado or other emergencies happen. It would be wise to keeps a mini-survival kit in your desk. With things like bottled water, hard candy, dried soup, tea, I even suggest at least one or two sternos, and any non-perishable eatable items. Along with a first aid kit.

Emergency Water Supply

(Information found on FEMA webpage)

Keep an emergency supply of drinking water in plastic containers. Commercially bottled drinking water is available. It stays pure for months and has the expiration date clearly marked on it.

There are several other sources of water if your water supply is turned off, water drained from the hot water tank (usually contains 30-60 gallons of usable water), clear water from the toilet flush-tank, if kept constantly clean. (Not the bowl!)

Melted ice cubes, canned fruits and vegetables juices, and liquid from canned goods.

1. If water is cloudy, smelly, or otherwise polluted, in strain it through a paper towel or several layers of clean cloth into a container order to remove any sediment or floating matter.

2. Water that is boiled vigorously for five full minutes will usually be safe from harmful bacterial contamination.

3. If boiling is not possible, strain the water as above and treat by adding ordinary liquid chlorine household bleach or tincture of iodine. Since liquid chlorine bleach loses strength over time, fresh bleach should be used as a water disinfectant. If the bleach is a year old the amount should be doubled. Two-year-old bleach should not be used as a water disinfectant.

4. Other chemical treatments for water purification also include halzone tablets, iodine tablets, or crystals. Mix thoroughly by stirring or shaking the

water in its container. Let it stand for 30 minutes. A slight chlorine odor should be detectable in the water, if not, repeat the dosage and let the water stand for an additional 15 minutes before using. Use an eye dropper to add the chlorine or the iodine to the water. Use it only for this purpose.

How to Prepare and Store Bottles of Purified Water

Keep drinking water safe from contamination by carefully storing in clean non-corrosive, tightly-covered containers. Use one-gallon containers, preferably made of heavy opaque plastic with screw-on-caps. Plastic milk bottles are not recommended. Sterilize the bottles.

> Number of drops to be added per quart of water:
>
> Chlorine should be clean not cloudy.
>
> Common household laundry bleach 2-3 drops.
>
> Tincture of iodine 3-6 drops.
>
> From medicine chest or first aid kit (2% chlorine) (rotate your iodine each year to ensure that it will work when you need it.)
>
> Emergency Water Supply
>
> 1. Wash bottles with soapy water, then rinse thoroughly.

2. Run about three quarts tap water into one of the containers, then add ¾ cup of bleach to the water.

3. Shake well, turning upside down a time or two so that the stopper will be sterilized also.

4. Let the mixture stand for two to three minutes, then pour it into the next container. You can use the same chlorinated water for several containers.

5. Fill the empty bottle with pure or purified water and seal it tightly, close with clean cap or stopper.

6. Label with "drinking water-purified," and the date of preparation.

7. Water purification tablets may also be used aid and are available in drug stores and sporting goods stores. They are recommended for your first aid kit. Four tablets will purify one filter

8. Some stored water may develop a disagreeable appearance, taste, or odor. These properties are not necessarily harmful. Inspect your water supply every few months to see whether the containers have leaked or other undesirable conditions have developed. Replace the water if it becomes contaminated.

Portable Water Purification Equipment

A high quality filter system should possess the following characteristics: light-weight, have fewer parts (less to go wrong) a fine pre-filter, a replaceable or clearable filter, tight, well-made pump high volume output, quick filtration, should screen out organisms over 0.5 microns (0.2 microns is best).

A system with all of these features may not be inexpensive, however, the cost will usually reflect reliability as well as technology of design. Always use a filter properly. Use clearest water available, allowing suspended matter to settle out. Use pre-filter is your system has one. Do not let outlet end of filter come in contact with contaminated water. Be sure vessel you're pumping into is clean.

Sanitize all bottles! ¼ cup Clorox to 1 quart water.

Emergency Heating, Cooking and Lighting

(Information found on www.survivalring.org)

HEATING

Coal stores well if kept in a dark place and away from moving air. Air speeds deterioration and breakdown, causing it to burn more rapidly. Coal may be stored in a plastic-lined pit or shield pit or in sheds, bags, boxes, or barrels and should be kept away from circulating air, light, and moisture. Cover it to lend protection from weather and sun.

WOOD

Hardwood such as apple, cherry, and other fruit woods are slow burning and sustain coal. Hardwoods are more difficult to burn than softer woods, thus requiring a supply of kindling. Soft woods such as pine and cedar are light weight and burn very rapidly, leaving ash and few coals for cooking. If you have a fireplace or wood/coal burning stove, you will want to store several cords of firewood.

Firewood is usually sold by the cord which is a neat pile that totals 128cubic feet. This pile is four feet wide, four feet high, and eight feet long. Some dealers sell wood by the ton. As a general rule of thumb, a standard cord of air dried dense hardwood weighs about two tons and provides as much heat as one ton of coal. Be suspicious of any alleged cord delivered in ½ or ¾ ton pickup truck.

For best results, wood should be seasoned (dried) properly, usually at least a year. A plastic tarp, wood planks, or other plastic or metal the sheeting over the woodpile is useful in keeping the wood dry. Other types of fuels are more practical to store and use than wood or coal. Newspaper logs make a good an inexpensive source of fuel. You may prepare the logs in the following manner:

> * Use about eight pages of newspaper and open flat.

> * Spread the stack, alternating the cut sides and folded sides.

* Place a 1" wood dowel or metal rod across one end and roll the paper around the rod very tightly. Roll it until there are 6-8 inches left to roll, then slip another 8 pages underneath the roll. Continue this diameter.

* With a fine wire, tie the roll on both ends. The Withdraw rod. Your newspaper log is ready to use. Four of these logs will burn about 1 hour.

* Propane is another excellent fuel for indoor use. Like kerosene, it produces carbon dioxide as it burns and is therefore not poisonous. It does not consume oxygen so be sure to crack a window when burning propane.

Stoves and small portable heaters are very economical, simple to use, and come the closet to approximating the type of convenience most of us are accustomed to using on a daily basis.

The storage of propane is governed by strict local laws. In this area you store up to 1 gallon inside a building and up to 60 gallons stored outside. If you store more than these amounts, you will need a special permit from the fire marshal.

The primary hazard in using propane is that it is heavier than air and if a leak occurs it may "pool" which can create an explosive atmosphere. Furthermore, basement natural gas heating units CANNOT be legally converted for propane use. Again, the vapors are heavier than air and form pockets." Ignition sources such as water heaters and electrical sources can cause an explosion.

White gas (Coleman fuel), Many families have camp stoves which burn Coleman fuel or white gasoline. These stoves are fairly easy to use and produce a great amount of heat. NEVER use a Coleman fuel stove indoors. It could be a fatal mistake to your entire family.

Never store fuel in the house or near a heater. Use a metal store cabinet which vented on top and bottom and can be locked.

Kerosene (also known as Range Oil No. 1) is the cheapest of all the storage fuels and is also very forgiving if you make a mistake. Kerosene is not as explosive as gasoline and Coleman fuel. Kerosene stores well for long periods of time by introducing some fuel additives, it ca be made to store even longer. However, do not store it in metal containers for extended time periods unless they are porcelain lined because the moisture in the kerosene will rust through the container causing the kerosene to leak out.

Most hardware stores and home improvement centers sell kerosene in five gallon plastic containers which store for many years. A 55 gallon drum stores in the backyard, or ten 5 gallon plastic containers will provide fuel enough to last an entire winter if used sparingly. Caution: To burn kerosene you will need a kerosene heater. There are many models and sizes to choose from but remember that you are not trying to heat your entire home. The larger the heater the more fuel you will have to store.

Most families should be able to get by on a heater that produces about 9,600 BTUs of heat, though kerosene heaters are made and will produce up to 25,000 to 30,000 BTUs. If you have the storage space to store the fuel required by these larger heaters they are excellent investments, but for most families the smaller heaters are more than adequate.

When selecting a kerosene heater be sure to get one that can double as a cooking surface and source of light. Then when you are forced to use it be sure to plan your meals so that they can be cooked when you are using the heater for heat, rather than wasting fuel used for cooking only. When kerosene burns it requires very little oxygen, compared to charcoal. You must crack a window about ¼ inch to allow enough oxygen to enter the room to prevent asphyxiation. During combustion, kerosene is not poisonous and is safe to use indoors.

To prevent possible fires you should always fill it outside. The momentary incomplete combustion during lighting and extinguishing of kerosene heaters can cause some unpleasant odors. To prevent these odors from lingering in your home normal operation a kerosene heater is practically odorless.

Charcoal

Never use a charcoal burning device indoors. When charcoal burns it is a voracious consumer of oxygen and will quickly deplete the oxygen supply in your little "home within a home." Furthermore, as it burns it produces vast amounts of carbon monoxide which is deadly poison. If you make the mistake of trying to heat your home by burning charcoal it could prove fatal to your entire family. Never burn charcoal indoors.

Cooking

To conserve your cooking fuel storage needs always do your emergency cooking in the most efficient manner possible. Don't boil more water that you need, extinguish the fire as soon as you finish, plan your meals ahead of time to consolidate as much cooking as possible, during the winter cook on top of your heating unit while heating your home, and cook in a pressure cooker or other fuel efficient containers as much as possible. Keep enough fuel to provide outdoor cooking for at least 7-10 days.

It is even possible to cook without using fuel at all. For example, to cook dry beans you can place them inside a pressure cooker with the proper amount of water and other ingredients needed and place it on your heat source until it comes up to pressure. Then turn the heat off, remove the pressure cooker and place inside a large box filled with newspapers, blankets, or other insulating materials. Leave it for two and a half hours and then open it, your meal will be done, having cooked for two and a half hours with no heat. If you do not have a large box in which to place it in the pressure cooker, simply wrap it in several blankets and place it in the corner.

Sterno fuel, a jelly petroleum product, is an excellent source of fuel for inclusion in your back pack as part of your 72 hour kit. Sterno is very light weight and easily ignited with a match or a spark from flint and steel but is not explosive. It is also safe for indoors. A Sterno stove can be purchased at any sporting goods store and will be retailed between three and eight dollars depending up on the model you choose. They fold up into a very small compact unit I deal for carrying in a pack. The fuel is readily available at all sporting goods stores and many drugstores. One can of sterno fuel about the diameter of a can of tuna fish and twice as high, will allow you to cook six meals if used frugally. Chafing dishes and fondue pots can also be used with sterno.

Sterno is not without some problems. It will evaporate very easily, even when the lid is securely fastened. If you use sterno in your 72 hour kit you should check it six to eight months to insure that it has not evaporated beyond the point of usage. Because of this problem it is not a good fuel for long time storage. It is very expensive fuel to use compared to other fuel available, but it is extremely convenient and portable.

Coleman fuel white gas, when used with a Coleman stove is another excellent and convenient fuel for cooking. It is not as portable nor as lightweight as sterno, but produces a much greater BTU value. Like sterno, Coleman fuel has a tendency to evaporate even when the container is tightly sealed so it is not a good fuel for long term storage. Unlike sterno, it is highly volatile, it will explode under the right conditions and should therefore never be stored in the home. Because of its highly flammable nature great care should always be exercised when lighting stoves and lanterns that may use Coleman fuel. Always store Coleman fuel in the garage or shed, outdoors.

Charcoal is the least expensive fuel per BTU that the average family can store. Remember that it must always be use out of doors because of the vast amounts of poisonous carbon monoxide it produces. Charcoal will store for extended periods of time if it is stored in air tight containers. It readily absorbs moisture from the surrounding air, so do not store it in the paper bags it comes in for more than a few months or it may be difficult to light. Transfer it to air tight metal or plastic containers and it will keep almost forever.

Fifty or sixty dollars' worth of charcoal will provide all the cooking fuel a family will need for an entire year if used sparingly. The Best time to buy briquettes are usually sold at a big discount. You will also want to store a small amount of charcoal lighter fluid or kerosene. Newspapers will also provide an excellent ignition source for charcoal when used in a funnel type of lighting device.

To light charcoal using newspaper use two or three sheets, crumpled up, and a#10 tin can. Cut both ends out of the can.

Punch holes every two inches around the lower edge of the can with a punch type can opener (for opening juice cans.) Set the can down so the punched holes are on the bottom. Place the crumpled newspaper in the bottom of the can and place the Charcoal briquettes on top of the newspaper. Lift the can slightly and light the newspaper. Prop a small rock under the bottom edge of the can to create a good draft. The briquettes will be ready to use in about 20-30 minutes. When the coals are ready remove the chimney and place them in your cooker. Never place burning charcoals directly on concrete or cement because the heat will crack it. A wheel barrel or old metal garbage can lid makes an excellent container for this type of fire.

One of nice things about charcoal is that you can regulate the heat you will receive from them. Each briquette will produce about 40 degrees of heat. If you are baking bread for example, and need 400 degrees of heat for your oven, simply use 10 briquettes.

To conserve heat and thereby get the maximum heat value from your charcoal you must learn to funnel the heat where you want it rather than letting it dissipate into the air around you. One excellent way to do this is to cook inside a cardboard oven. Take a cardboard box, about the size of an orange crate, and cover it with aluminum foil inside and out. Be sure that the shiny side is visible so that the maximum reflectivity is achieved. Turn the box on its side so that the opening is no longer on the Top But is on the side. Place some small bricks or other non-combustible material inside upon which you can rest a cookie sheet about two or three inches about the bottom the box. Please ten burning Charcoal briquettes between the bricks (If you need 400 degrees), place the support for your cooking vessels, and then place your bread pans or whatever else you are using on top of the cookie sheet. Prop a foil covered cardboard lid over the open side, leaving a large crack for air to get in (Charcoal needs a lot of air to burn) and bake your bread, cake, cookies, etc. just like you would in your regular oven. Your results will amaze you.

To make your own Charcoal, select twigs, limbs, and branches of fruit, nut and other hardwood trees. Black walnuts and peach or apricot pits may also be used. Cut wood into desired size, place in a large can which has a few holes punched in it, put a lid on the can and place the can and a hot fire. When the flames from the holes in the can turn yellow – red, remove the can from the fire and allow it to cool. Store the briquettes in a moisture – proof contender. Burn charcoal only in a well ventilated area. Wood and coal. Many wood and coal burning stoves are made with cooking surface. These excellent to use indoors during the winter because you may already be using it to heat the home. In the summer, however, they are unbearably hot and are simply not practical cooking appliances for indoor use. If you choose to build a campfire on the ground outside be sure to use caution and follow all the rules for safety. Little children and even many adults, are not aware of the tremendous dangers that open fires may pose.

Kerosene

Many kerosene heaters will also double as a cooking unit. In fact, it is probably a good idea to not purchase a kerosene heater that cannot be used to cook on as well. Follow the same precautions for cooking over kerosene as was discussed under the section on heating your home with kerosene.

Propane

Many families have propane camp stoves. These are the most convenient and easy to use of all emergency cooking appliances available. They may be used indoors or out. As with other emergency fuel sources, cook with a pressure cooker whenever possible to conserve fuel.

Lighting

Most of the alternatives require a fire or flame, so use caution. More home fires are caused by improper usage of fires used for light than for any other purpose. Especially use extra caution with children and flame. Teach them the proper safety procedures to follow under emergency conditions. Allow them to practice these skills under proper adult supervision now, rather than waiting until an emergency strikes.

Cyalume sticks are the safest form indoor lighting available but very few people even know what they are. Cyalume sticks can be purchased at most sporting goods stores for about $2 per stick. They are a plastic stick about four inches in length and a half inch in diameter. To activate them, simply bend them until the glass tube inside them breaks, then shake to mix the chemicals inside and it will grow a bright green light for up to eight hours. Cyalume is the only form of light that is safe to turn on inside a home after an earthquake. One of the great dangers after a serious earthquake is caused by ruptured natural gas lines. If you flip on a light switch or even turn on a flashlight you run the risk of causing an explosion. Cyalume will not ignite natural gas. Cyalume sticks are so safe that a baby can even use them for a tether.

Flashlights are excellent for most types of emergencies except in situations where ruptured natural gas lines may be present. Never turn a flashlight on or off if there is any possibility of ruptured gas lines. Go outside first, turn it on or off, then enter the building. The three main problems with relying upon flashlights is that they give light to very small areas, the batteries run down fairly quickly during use, and batteries do not store well for extended time periods. Alkaline batteries store the best if stored in a cool location and in an airtight container. These batteries should be expected to store for three to five years. Many manufacturers are now printing a date on the package indicating the date through which the batteries should be good. When stored under ideal conditions the shelf life will be much longer than that indicated. Lithium batteries will store for about twice as long as alkaline

If you use flashlights be sure to use krypton or halogen light bulbs in them because they last much longer and give off several times more light than regular flashlight bulbs on the same energy consumption. Store at least two or three extra bulbs in a place where they will not be crushed or broken.

Candles

Every family should have a large supply of candles. Three hundred sixty five candles, or one per day is not too many. The larger the better. Fifty hour candles are available in both solid and liquid form. White or light colored candles burn brighter than dark candles. Tallow candles burn brighter, longer, and are fairly smoke free when compared to wax candles. Their lighting ability can be increased by placing an aluminum foil reflector behind them or by placing them in front of a mirror. However, candles are extremely dangerous indoors because of high fire danger, especially around children. For this reason be sure to store several candle lanterns or broad based candle holders. Be sure to store a goodly supply of wooden matches, save your candle ends for emergency use. Votive candles set in empty jars will burn up to 15 hours. Non-candles (plastic dish and paper wicks) and a bottle of salad oil will provide hundreds of hours of candle light.

Trench candles can be used as fireplace fuel or as a candle for light. To make trench candles:
1. Place a narrow strip of cloth or twisted string (for wick) on the edge of a stack of 6-10 newspapers.
2. Roll the papers very tightly, leaving about ¾ of wick extending at each end.

3. Tie the roll firmly with string or wire at 2-4 intervals.
4. With a small saw cut about I inch above each tie and pull the cut sections into cone shape. Pull the center string in each piece toward the top of the cane to serve as a wick.
5. Met paraffin in a large saucepan set inside a larger pan of hot water. Soak the pieces of candles in the paraffin for about 2 minutes.
6. Remove the candles and place on a newspaper to dry.

Kerosene lamps are excellent sources of light and will burn for approximately 45 hours on a quart of fuel. They burn bright and are inexpensive to operate. The main problem with using them is failure to properly trim the wicks and using the wrong size chimney. Wicks should be trimmed in an arch, a "V," "A" or straight across the top. Failure to properly trim and maintain wicks will result in smoke and poor light.

Aladdin type lamps that use a circular wick and mantle do not need trimming and produces much more light (and heat) than conventional kerosene lamps. These lamps, however, produce a great amount of heat, getting up to 750 degrees F. If placed within 36 inches of any combustible object such as wooden cabinets, walls, etc. Charring can occur. Great caution should therefore be exercised to prevent accidental fires.

Propane and Coleman lanterns

Camp lanterns burning Coleman fuel or propane make excellent
Sources of light. Caution should be used in filling and lighting Coleman lanterns because the fuel is highly volatile and a flash type fire is easy to set off. Always fill them outside. Propane, on the other hand, is much safer. It is not as explosive and does not burn quite as hot. A double mantle lantern gives off as much light as two 100-watt light bulbs. Either propane or Coleman fuel type lanterns are very reliable and should be an integral part of your preparedness program. Be sure to store plenty of extra mantles and matches.

Store lots of wooden matches (1,000-2,000 is not too many). Also store butane cigarette lighters to light candles, lanterns and fireplaces. It would be a good idea for everyone to have a personal fire

building kit with at least six different ways to start
a fire.

Above all, your home and family must be
protected from the ravages of fire by your actions.
Study the instructions for any appliances used for a
heating, cooking, or lighting and understand there
features as well as their limitations.

Don't go to sleep with any invented burning device
in your home. Your family might not wake up.

Whatever you store, store it safely and legally. In
an emergency, survival may cause you to make
decisions that are questionable with regard to
safety.

Become educated to the inherent hazards of your
choices and make a decision based on as much
verifiable information as possible. You and your
family's lives will depend on it.

Consider carefully how you will provide fuel for
your family for heating, cooking, and lighting
during times of emergencies. Next to food, water,
and shelter, energy is the most important item you
can store.

The Herbal Survival Guidebook

PSALM 24:1-2 (NIV)

Psalm 24

Of David. A psalm.

[1] **The earth is the LORD's, and everything in it,
the world, and all who live in it;
[2] for he founded it on the seas
and established it on the waters.**

CHAPTER 2

THE FOODS YOUR FAMILY WIIL NEED

1. Your family will need.

2. The names of family members.

3. The ages of family members.

4. 1 pound per person of: Grains, wheat, flour, corn meal, oats, rice, and pasta.

5. 1 pound per person of: legumes, dry beans, lima beans, soy beans, split peas, lentils, and dry soup mixes.

6. 1 pound per person of: sugars, honey, pure cane, natural brown sugar, molasses, natural jams/jellies.

7. 1 pound per person of: baking powder, baking soda, yeast, salt, and vinegar.

8. Gallons of fats and oils, vegetable oils, canola, olive oil, soy oil, organic mayonnaise, and peanut butter.

9. Milks, dry milk, evaporated milk, powdered soy milk, rice milk, shelf milk, Babies formula.

10. Gallons of water.

11. Other essentials, dried fruits, natural hard candies, canned

dried meats, dried and canned natural powdered juices.

These items should be kept in an airtight plastic storage bin and mark with the date and year stored as well as the contents.

Remember to always check on your food for the dates of expiration, and update them as they expire. Hebrews, for the earth which drinkethin the rain that cometh oft upon it, and

bringeth forth herbs meat for them by whom it is dressed, receiveth blessings from GOD.

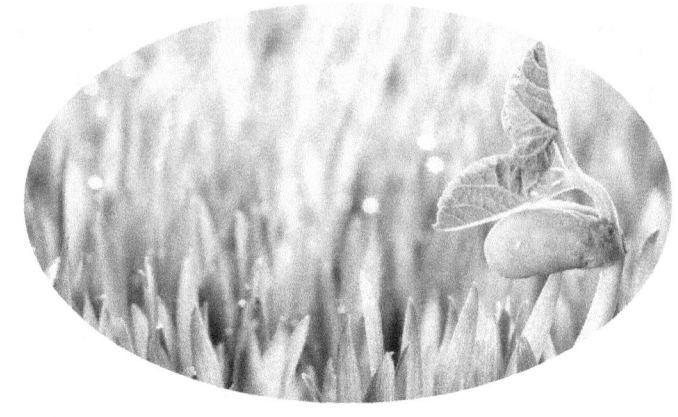

CHAPTER 3

THE EMERGENCY HERBAL MEDICINE CHEST

1. Rosemary, Chamomile, Valerian, Passion Flower, and Skullcap, are the times herbs for insomnia.

2. Lemon balm, Lemongrass, Ginseng, Kava Kava, Chamomile, and St. John's Wort are the top herbs for Stress relief and tension.

3. Ginger tea, Peppermint tea, Fennel tea, Aloe Vera juice, and Catnip herbs are the top herbs for indigestion, gas, heartburn, and upset stomach relief.

4. Aloe Vera juice wash, Eyebright, Bilberry wash, Dandelion Wash, Echinacea or Goldenseal wash, Witch Hazel solution, and Parsley wash are the top herbs for eye infections, inflammation, redness and dry eyes.

5. Clove oil, Tea tree oil and Myrrh Gum are the top herbs for toothaches, and gum problems.

6. Skullcap, Peppermint or Wintergreen oil rubs, Feverfew, Comfrey compresses, Rosemary or Lavender tea, White Willow Bark, and Lemon balm are the top herbs for pain, cramping and headache relief.

7. Marshmallow, Echinacea, Aloe Vera gel, Tea Tree Oil, Plantain Oil, or compresses and Comfrey ointment are the top herbs for itching, insect bites, and rashes.

8. Pau De Arco, Witch Hazel, Aloe Vera gel, Tea Tree oil, Lavender Leaf or oil, heal all. Comfrey salves are the top herbs for cuts, burns, wounds and scrapes.

9. Licorice Root, Echinacea, Wild Cherry Bark, Peppermint, Goldenseal, and Aloe Vera juice are

the top herbs for coughs, colds, flu, and sore throats.

10. Peppermint, Mullein, Lavender, Eucalyptus, Ginger, Echinacea, Goldenseal, and Wintergreen are the top herbs for viruses, chest congestion, earaches, and flu.

THE HERBAL FIRST AID MEDICINE KIT

Remember the first aid is just a band aid until adequate medical attention can be found. However, it is good to learn as much as you can should emergencies arise. Especially when crisis like a hurricane, flood, or any type of disaster hits. As soon as the crisis is over, follow up on any serious injuries or illnesses with a qualified physician.

Aloe, break off an aloe leaf and apply the gel to soothe minor burns, sunburns, cutes, scrapes and scalds. Aloe tissue regenerative properties and will help heal all wounds.

Arnica, arnica cream, gel, or oil or even pill form can be used on or for bruises or sprains where the skin is not broken. It can also help to ease pain and discomfort when taken orally. Arnica should be you sparingly because it can become extremely toxic is high doses.

Calendula cream, is a good antiseptic and antifungal for many things. It has a great and speedy healing process.

Clove oil, clove oil is a great antiseptic for cuts, bruises, it is also good for treating tooth aches and other diseases. It should however always be cut with a carrier Oil when used on the skin. Severe allergic reactions could occur.

Making your own compresses, keep squares of gauze, cheesecloth, or flannel material on hand to make compresses. Use comfrey, Witch Hazel or Arnica for Sprains, use St John's Wort or heal all for those deep nasty cuts, use Aloe, Lavender, or Comfrey for Burns.

Ginger, Chamomile, Raspberry, and Peppermint, are all good to either Chew on or make an herbal tea and drink for morning sickness, nausea, or motion sickness.

Eucalyptus oil, is good as and inhalant for colds, mix with Olive oil, can't be used for a chest rub, it is great for relieving sinus headaches, coughs, and respiratory infections.

St. John's Wort, is great for calming nerves, headaches, helping you to sleep. If mixed with olive oil, it cannot be used for minor burns and sunburns.

Slippery Elm Bark, is used in powder form for making poultices for drawing out splinters and bringing boils to a head.

Tea Tree Oil is by far the best antiseptic and antifungal agent, and can be used for wounds, fungus, and minor infections, etc.

Witch Hazel Extract, can be purchased in any health food store, this can be used to treat minor burns, cuts, sunburns, insect bites and scrapes. It can also be used to stop nosebleeds by applying it to the nasal passages.

The syrup of ipecac is a standard remedy which promotes vomiting and should only be used in certain types of poisoning.

Flower rescue remedy, is used for emotional trauma for all ages. Flower essences usually works quickly and effectively on many symptoms ranging from hyperventilation, panic attacks, hysteria, etc. It can be taken orally or can be rubbed on the temples and wrists. It has an immediate calming effect. If you use an extract, it will keep its potency for several years if stored in a dark cool place.

Three very important essential oils to have are and Peppermint for upset stomach, or to rub on the temples to stay awake. Tea Tree oil, which is known as first aid kit in the bottle because of its strong antifungal, antiseptic, and antibiotic properties with the ability to help with infections, wounds, burns, cold sores, lesions, fungus, earaches and so much more. Remember to mix it with equal parts of olive oil, because the Tea Tree oil is very strong. You only need to use a little, this oil goes a long way.

Good antimicrobials are, Echinacea, Goldenseal, Oregon Grape Root, Myrrh Gum, Garlic, Calendula, Chamomile, Gentian, and Grape Seed

Extract.

Good astringents are, Horse Tail, Geranium, Rose, Alum, Yarrow, Witch Hazel, Yellow Dock, and St. John's Wort.

LUKE 11:9-10 (NIV)

[9] "So I say to you: Ask and it will be given to you; seek and
you will find; knock and the door will be opened to
you. [10] For everyone who asks receives; the one who seeks
finds; and to the one who knocks, the door will be opened.

CHAPTER 4

TEACHING YOURSELF FIRST AID

I can never explain how important it is to have a
FIRST AID KIT But everyone should take a first
aid and a CPR course.

**But there are some helpful training to start you
on your way.**
1. The supplies you will need our sterile gauze,
lint dressings, (about four inches by four inches in
size) wound dressings, like strips of clean cotton
cloths.

2. Bandages, all shapes and sizes.

3. Cotton wool.

4. And assortment of adhesive dressings.

5. and assortment of adhesive tapes.

6. Antiseptic, alcohols, peroxide, Witch Hazel, green slopes.

7. Blood pressure kit.

8. Scissors.

9. Tongue depressors (which can be used for tourniquets).

10. Pocket Knife.

11. Medical and Herbal First Aid Books.

HEBREWS 11:3NEW INTERNATIONAL VERSION (NIV)

[3] By faith we understand that the universe was formed at God's command, so that what is seen was not made out of what was visible.

The Collapsed Patient

This may be your first time trying to help a person who has collapsed/fainted. First you must be calm and quickly assess the situation. There may be several reasons why this person has passed out. It could be seizures, a heart attack, stroke, fear or some other medical reasons.

In case of a person collapsing there are two most important things you can do, first you must check the respiration and circulation.

Respiration

It is very essential to make sure that the individual is breathing and that the airway is clear. If the brain is not getting enough oxygen for more than a few minutes then irreversible damage can occur.

Circulation

The pulses should be checked at the wrist and on the neck, directly under the ear. First check for the radial and then the carotid artery. If there is no breathing and no pulse, then cardio-pulmonary resuscitation (CPR) should be started.

Cardio-Pulmonary Resuscitation

This is the life saving techniques that everyone should know. These classes are offered at the Red Cross or Community Colleges, etc.

But just in case let's pretend that the person who has fainted is alone, and you cannot call 911 because the phones are out. Here are two very important points.

1. The airway must be clear, otherwise there is a risk of blowing a foreign object further down the airway, and possibly choking the individual. (Remember that the individual could have collapsed from choking on food or candy, etc.)

2. External chest compression must not be done if there is a pulse or heartbeat. The danger is that beating a heart that may be already weak could stop the heart from beating completely.

Artificial Ventilation

The first thing to do is make sure that the individual is lying on a firm surface. However, if the patient is a casualty case and a neck or spinal problem is suspected try not to move, or move as little as possible.

Nest, tilt the head back slightly, in order to open the airway. Check immediately for a pulse. If there is a pulse then chest compression should not be performed.

A handkerchief or a form of material must be placed over the patient's mouth. (This protects you and the patient) then with a full breath in, open the mouth fully and seal it around the patient's mouth. Blow, watching the rise of the chest. As it rises, stop blowing, physically turn and watch it go down again as you take another breath to fill your lungs. Give 4 quick breaths like this then check the pulse. If the pulse is present then you should do 16 ventilations per minute.

Chest Compression

I must urge you to take a CPR course, there is no substitute for seeing the actual training. Kneel beside the patient. If and only if there is no pulse should this be done? Feel for the angle at the bottom of the rib cage at the top of the abdomen. Place the heel of the hand on the sternum, two finger breaths above the angle. Then place the palm of the other hand above it. Keep the elbows straight and lean forward to compress the chest. An adult's chest wall should be compressed by 1 inch, a child's by ½ inch.

15 compression at a rate of 80 bpm's, should be given. This is slightly more than compression per second. After 15 compressions the patient should be given two ventilations. Check the pulse. Repeat the cycle until heartbeat and respiration start, or until help and relief arrive.

Recovery Signs

The patient starts to lose the cyanosis. This means that oxygen is reaching the tissue. The pulse returns. The breathing restarts, often preceded by a groan.

Recovery Position

Once the patient starts to show some recovery signs, you need to place them in a recovery position. Kneel beside the patient and gently turn their body. Draw the other arm across the chest and cross the farther ankle over the one nearest you. Gently roll the patient towards you, taking care to avoid injury to their head or spine. Once you have moved them over towards you, tilt their head to ensure that the airway remains open. Then bend their arm and knee nearest to you so that they will not roll over.

When an Epileptic Fit Occurs

Epilepsy is best regarded as the symptoms of some underlying brain dysfunctions, which causes gross misbehavior of the brain cells, either at a specific place, or more widely. This misbehavior causes physical consequences, like loss of consciousness, or loss of muscle control, and possible convulsions.

There are several types of epilepsy. Traditionally, two types of fits were distinguished,

Petit Mal: Absence and mood related fits, with no physical manifestation.

Grand Mal: Major fits, with loss of consciousness, muscle spasms, and after effects.

Grand Mal is the name given to major form.

There are different stages. The precursor may be that the individual may experience and aura, a set of symptoms which forewarn him/her that an attack is about to start. This may take the form of peculiar taste, smells, sounds and or visuals.

The tonic phase follows. Here the individual falls, become stiff and the face starts to go red, pale or even purple.

The clonic phase occurs when the individual starts to shake, often violently. The face may grimace, their breathing may be slow, there may be salivation from their mouth, and incontinence may occur. The relaxation phase follows as the convulsions start to pass over. The patient drifts into sleep. This may last for a few minutes or several hours.

How to Manage

The first thing is to clear things away from the surroundings area so that the patient does not injure him/herself. A cushion or some sort of pad should be placed under the head. The individual may be carrying an epilepsy card which will inform you of the type of problem they may suffer from, and who to contact.

You should never attempt to put anything into their mouth. The individual I not likely to swallow their own tongue, so you are more likely to cause injury to their mouth or injury to yourself.

Remember to keep calm, do not panic. Do not restrain the person. Make sure you protect their head, talk calmly to the person and reassure them that everything will be alright.

Pay attention to how long, the seizure lasts, if it lasts for more than 5 minutes then call for an ambulance. Once the seizure starts to subside, put the person into a comfortable position and stay with them until they have fully recovered. If possible you should call a relative or friend so that they can the person to the hospital. Check to see if the person has their medication. And help them to take it at that time.

Note: Some people may have to take a rectal medication to break their fit cycle, as the patient may have more than 1 seizure, or it may last for longer than 5 minutes. If this is the case, this medication should be given by a trained person.

When a Person is Choking

I happen to be a person that chokes very easily, especially if I am eating and someone makes me laugh. And since I had the stroke it got worse. Choking usually occurs when some foreign substance, like food, saliva, water, etc. is inhaled into the larynx. Laughing, inhaling quickly, coughing, and sneezing with something in the mouth can be the cause.

The individual should be encouraged to cough, I find that if they can talk, that is a start. They should be bent over and slapped between the shoulder blades. This should be done up to 4 times. Check the mouth again for the object.

The abdominal thrust method should be used if this fails. This should only be used if the other methods have failed. Stand behind the individual and put an arm around them. Clench the fist and place it in the middle of the abdomen, about the umbilicus. The closed fist should be so positioned that the phone knuckle is against the individual's abdominal wall. The fist is grasped with the other and both are pulled in a sudden thrust. This can be done up to 4 times. Clear out the mouth after each attempted procedure.

Asthma Attacks

The asthmatic should always have an inhaler in their possession. They should be asked if they have their inhaler and if they take any medication or herbal supplements for their asthma. It they have these items, they should be able to take it themselves or you may have to administer these items to them very gingerly. But, if there is no improvement, then medical help should be sought instantly. People still die from asthma attacks, so treatment should not be delayed. However, in case emergency i.e. the phones are dead, or one help cannot get to you fast, help them patient as much as possible. To get them to breath easily can be done by deep breathing exercises. This will relax them and help them to breath or evenly.

Nosebleeds

There are a lot of different ideas about stopping nosebleeds. The nose must be pinched on the fleshy part below the bony part of the nose. The individual should be allowed to sit forward over a basin and the pressure should be maintained for at least 10 minutes. The pressure should then be gradually released.

Chest Pains

Central chest pain, especially with radiation into the neck or down the arms must be assumed to be due to myocardial ischemia until proved otherwise. The patient must be allowed into the half sitting position with the head, knees and shoulders supported by cushions. They should be encouraged to try to relax while help is obtained urgently. Tight clothing should be released. Deep breathing should be administered. Help should be called immediately, however it for any reason you cannot call someone 1/2 of an aspirin could be given to help ease some of the pain. Make sure that the patient can take aspirin.

Bone Fracture Home Remedy

When a bone in the body breaks or cracks it is called a fracture. There are two types of fractures, closed or simple, when the skin that covers the bone remains intact or it's open or compound when not bone breaks the skin. When a fracture occurs, it causes terrible pain and tenderness in the area fractured, along with swelling the appearance of some blood under the skin and numbness, tingling or paralysis below the injured area.

When a person fractures an arm or leg, he or she can lose the pulse below the fracture. Fractures are more common in Young children and in older adults. As we grow older, our bones get weaker and more fragile, and they take more time to heal themselves. A fracture requires professional attention, what we offer here are recommendations that will aid in healing after the bone has been set.

I Suggest

---

1. Eat half a pineapple every day until it is completely healed. It contains bromelain, and enzyme that helps to reduce swelling and inflammation. Do not eat canned or processed pineapples. If you don't like pineapples, take the supplement Bromelain. It has the same effect as pineapple.

2. It is very important to regain bone strength as soon as possible to avoid future injuries and two insure a solid bone fusion. Went recommend that you take this.

3. Do not eat red meat, and avoid drinking colas and all products containing caffeine.

4. Avoid eating foods with preservatives, they contain phosphorus which can lead to bone lost.

5. Take Boron, it is important for the health and healing of the bone.

6. Take Calcium, magnesium, potassium. They are essential to repair bone damage and to maintain a good muscle and heart condition.

7. Take Zinc, it helps repair tissue damage.

• Calcium Information

Essential calcium information for osteoporosis treatment, arthritis pain relief, to prevent bone disease, to improve bone density, back pain relief and promoting healthy strong bones.

DEUTERONOMY 6:24 (NIV)

[24] The LORD commanded us to obey all these decrees and to fear the LORD our God, so that we might always prosper and be kept alive, as is the case today.

There are some sites that can help you with free CPR and emergency training online, also sites that give basic medical information.

---

http://www.emergencyuniversity.com

1-877-REDCROSS has some free courses available to groups.

http://www.first-aid-product.com

http://www.training.fema.gov

http://www.survivalring.org/index.htm

http://ynhh.org/pediatrics/emergencies/first_aid.html

http://www.engenderhealth.org/ip/index/html

http://depts.washington.edu/learncpr

http://www.nlm.nih.gov/medlineplus

The Herbal Survival Guidebook

http://www.healthcarefreeware.com

http://www.healthy.net

http://www.safetycentral.com

The Herbal Survival Guidebook

PSALM 34:18-19 (NIV)

[18] The LORD is close to the brokenhearted
and saves those who are crushed in spirit.
[19] The righteous person may have many troubles,
but the LORD delivers him from them all;

Herbal First Aid Books and Sites

http://www.herbnet.com

http://www.westernbotanicals.com

http://wellnessmama.com/3516/natural-first-aid-kit

http://www.herbs-home-remedies.com/herbal-first-aid-for-the-home.html

http://www.herb-health-guide.com/first-aid-herbs-2.html

https://www.richters.com

http://naturalnurse.com

http://www.herbsociety-stu.org

http://www.home-remedies-for-you.com

http://www.vedicsociety.org

The Herbal Survival Guidebook

http://www.natural-homeremedies.org

http://draxe.com/the-top-14-herbs-of-the-bible

http://www.renewalofthespiritinstitute.com/

ABOUT THE AUTHOR

Dr. Donia Gonzales-Copeland MA. DPC.

I am the founder of Renewal of the Spirit Institute & Wholistic Center.

I hold a Doctorate in Pastoral counseling and certifications in Herbology, drug and alcohol counseling, aroma-therapy, prayer meditations, Healing Touch Therapy, Creative Healing Art Therapy, dream analysis & relaxation.

The wife and mother of four grown children, I have six grandchildren, and great grandchildren. I am a retire school councilor a stroke survivor and an herbalist since birth. i am now working on my new path. God Bless all who read this.

Email: renewalof48@yahoo.com

www.renewalofthespiritinstitute.com/

The Herbal Survival Guidebook

www.ingramcontent.com/pod-product-compliance
Lightning Source LLC
Chambersburg PA
CBHW071355310526
45790CB00017B/774